HOMEMADE HAND SANITIZER

Best Sanitizer Recipes for a Hygienic Lifestyle

Albert Leinstein

Homemade Hand Sanitizer - Albert Leinstein

Copyright © 2020 Albert Leinstein

All rights reserved

TABLE OF CONTENTS

Introduction — 2

Chapter 1 - Basic Hygiene — 4

Chapter 2 - The Basic of Hand Sanitizer — 19

Chapter 3 - Hand Sanitizer Recipes — 34

Chapter 4 - Homemade Disinfectant Wipes — 49

Conclusion — 71

Homemade Hand Sanitizer - Albert Leinstein

INTRODUCTION

First off, I would like to thank you for choosing *Homemade Hand Sanitizer: Best Sanitizer Recipes for a Hygienic Lifestyle*. I hope that you find the book informative and educational.

It is important that everybody, all over the world, every day practices good hygiene. Making sure you follow good hygienic practices helps to reduce your chances of getting sick and reduces the spread of communicable diseases. If history teaches us anything, it's that we never know when a disease may appear and begin spreading across the world. Unfortunately, everybody across the world doesn't have access to healthy hygienic practices like those in developed nations. This means that diseases tend to spread more easily in those countries. That said, diseases can still get a foothold in developed nations as well, but you can do your part by making sure you are clean and don't spread the disease.

This book is here to help you with that by providing you with information on basic hygiene and sanitization. The first thing we will go over is basic hygiene. While we all were taught basic handwashing and hygienic practices in kindergarten, it seems we could all use a refresher in the right way to wash our hands. It's amazing what washing your hands can do to prevent illnesses and the like.

Then we will go over the basics of hand sanitizer. Everybody loves to turn to hand sanitizer to help them kill off germs. Hand sanitizer is a great thing to have, but do you know how or why it is helpful? You will after this, and you will also learn the proper ways to use it because you can use it too much.

Next, we will go over a few different recipes to make your own hand sanitizer. There may be times when you can't find any sanitizer in the store, or you simply want to know exactly what goes into your sanitizer. These recipes will help you out for whatever reason.

Lastly, you will find several recipes to make your own disinfectant wipes. These can get pretty expensive when you buy them, and like most things, you can make them yourself for a lot less. Disinfectant wipes are also a great cleaning product to have in the home.

With all of this in mind, let's begin.

CHAPTER 1: BASIC HYGIENE

Washing your hands is one of the best ways to protect yourself and your family from getting sick. We are going to look at when and how you should wash your hands so that you and your family can remain healthy.

Making sure we keep our hands clean is the best way to make sure you don't spread germs or get sick. A lot of conditions and diseases are spread because people don't keep their hands clean. In this chapter, and throughout the book, you will see the words microbes and germs. Microbe refers to "all tiny living organisms that may or may not cause disease." Germs, or pathogens, are forms of microbes that can cause the development of diseases.

When to Wash Your Hands

There are times when you should wash your hands to make sure you don't spread germs around. There are also certain times of the year where you may want to wash your hands more often than you normally would. These times tend to be during the winter months when the cold and flu are the most active. The best times to make sure you wash your hands are:

- After your touch garbage of any kind

- After you have handled your pet's food or treats
- After you have touched any type of animal waste, animal feed, or animal
- After you have sneezed, coughed, or blow your nose
- After you have changed diapers or cleaned up a child who has just used the bathroom
- After you use the bathroom
- Before and after you treat a wound or cut
- Before and after you have cared for a person who is sick with vomiting or diarrhea
- Before you eat food
- Before, during, and after fixing food
- After you get off of public transit, cab, or other ride share
- After playing or working outdoors
- Before and after changing contact lenses

These are obviously not the only times you should wash your hands. Anytime your hands appear dirty, or you have been handling something that could have germs on it, you should wash your hands or use hand sanitizer. You should also make sure that you wash your hands several times during the day while at work. The CDC says that the average office worker's desk has more germs on it than the toilet seat. You should also wash your hands whenever you shake another person's hand since hand-to-hand contact is one of the most common ways that germs are spread.

Properly Washing Your Hands

One of the easiest things that you do in life is washing your hands. Having clean hands is able to stop the spread of germs within your home, workplace, and community. There are five steps that you should use every time you wash your hands.

1. Begin by wetting your hands with clean, running water (cold or warm), turn the tap off, and then apply soap.

The reason you want to use clean, running water is that if you simply place your hands in a container of standing water, you aren't cleaning them because the water has already been contaminated. You should always use clean, running water. However, if you have to wash your hands in non-potable water, it can still help to improve your health. Basically, it's better than nothing. It has been found that the temperature of the water doesn't have much to do with affecting the microbe removal. People often have the thought process of, "Warm or hot water would be better because heat kills bacteria," but, to get the temperature of the water to a level that would kill pathogens would end up burning you. However, warmer will create more skin irritation and is more costly environmentally. Keep the water cold or on the cooler side will help to save energy and water consumption.

Turning the faucet off after you have wet your hands will help to save water, and there isn't enough information to prove that a significant number of germs are spread from the faucet to your hands.

Using soap when washing your hands works a lot better than simply using water because the surfactants that the soap has helped to bring off the microbes and soil that are on your hand. People also have a tendency to wash more thoroughly when they have soap, which helps to remove more germs.

To date, studies have found that there aren't any additional health benefits for consumers, and this does not include healthcare professionals, to use soaps that contain antibacterial ingredients when compared to plain soap. This caused the FDA to issue a statement in September of 2016 that several of the most common ingredients used in "antibacterial" soaps, which includes triclosan, weren't any better than soaps that did not contain them, and this left companies having to remove them from their products or simply not market them towards the general population. This does not include antibacterial products that you are used by healthcare professionals.

2. Work the soap into a lather by rubbing your hands together so that they are covered with soap. Make sure that you lather the backs of the hands, under your nails, and between each finger.

When you lather and scrub your hands, it will create friction, which will help to lift up microbes, dirt, and grease from the skin. Microbes live all over your hands, but they tend to be more concentrated under your nails, so it is important that you scrub the entire hand.

3. Do this for at least 20 seconds. If you want to make sure you do it long enough, hum through "happy birthday" twice.

Figuring out the best length of time to wash your hands is hard because only a few studies about the impacts of changing handwashing time have been dome. Of the studies that have been done, almost all of them have found a lower number of microbes present on the skin, only a few of which may cause illness, and there are no measured impacts on health. Simply reducing how many microbes are on your skin doesn't necessarily mean it will improve your health. The correct amount of time to wash your hands is also probably dependant on many other factors, which include the amount and type of soil that you have on your hands and where you are when washing them.

For example, surgeons tend to have a higher chance of being in contact with germs that cause diseases and are at a greater risk of spreading diseases or infections to others, so that means they need to wash for a longer period of time than somebody cooking lunch at home. Nonetheless, they have found that washing for about 15 to 30 seconds will remove more germs than washing for less time.

This is a lot of organizations and countries that recommend you wash for about 20 seconds.

4. Rinse the soap off of your hands completely.

The soap and friction you created in the last step helps to lift off the microbes, dirt, and grease from the skin so that you are able to rinse them off of your hands. When you rinse the soap away, it will minimize irritation to the skin. Since hands are able to become recontaminated if you rinse them in a container of standing water that may have been contaminated from previous use, you should use clean, running water. While there are some people who recommend drying with paper towels and using them to turn the faucet off, it doesn't do much and can lead to a waste of paper towels and water.

5. Dry your hands off using a clean towel or allow them to air dry.

Germs are able to be transferred more easily to and from hands that are wet. This means that hands need to be dried off after washing them. However, it is still unclear what the best way to dry your hands is because there aren't a lot of studies about it, and the results tend to conflict with one another. Also, most studies compare the overall amount of microbes, and not just the disease-causing germs, that are present on the hands following different drying methods. Studies have shown that using a clean towel or air drying methods tend to work the best.

Why You Need to Wash Your Hands?

While this may seem obvious, especially after what we have talked about so far, it is important to make sure we understand the extreme importance of washing our hands. Hands touch everything, which means they are constantly coming in contact with some type of germ. These germs can cause people to get sick.

Feces from animals or people is one of the mains sources of germs like the norovirus,

Salmonella, and E. coli 0157 that all cause diarrhea, and it is able to spread respiratory infections like hand-foot-mouth disease and adenovirus. All of these germs are able to get on our hands after a person changes a diaper or uses the toilet, but you can also come in contact with it in less obvious ways. Handling things like raw meats that invisible amounts of animal feces on them. Just a gram of human feces, which what a paper clip weights, can hold one trillion germs. These germs can then get onto our hands if you touch any object that contains germs because somebody sneezed or coughed on it, or a contaminated object touched it. Whenever germs get on your hands, and you don't wash them off, they can then be passed to other people, which can make them sick.

Viruses and bacteria are extremely easy to transmit through most everything that you touch. It's pretty much impossible to avoid germs that could attack your immune system on a daily basis. This is why you need to be on the defensive.

Washing your hands helps to prevent illness and the spread of infectious diseases because washing your hands gets rid of germs. The reason this helps to prevent infections is that:

- People tend to touch their mouth, eyes, and noses without noticing they are doing it. This gives germs a quick route into the body, making the person sick.

- Germs on unwashed hands can easily enter drinks and foods while people consume or cook them. Germs are able to multiply in some types of drinks and foods, under the right conditions, and then make other sick.

- Germs on unwashed hands are able to be transferred to other objects, such as toys, handrails, or tabletops, and then transferred to other people.

- Getting rid of germs by washing your hand will, therefore, help to prevent respiratory infections and diarrhea and can help prevent eye and skin infections.

When people are taught proper handwashing techniques helps them and the communities to remain healthy. When handwashing education is shared in a community, it can:

- Reduce the days missed at school due to gastrointestinal illness by 29 to 57 percent.

- Reduce respiratory illnesses, such as the common cold, in the general population by 16 to 21 percent.

- Reduce diarrheal illnesses in those with suppressed immune systems by 58 percent.

- Reduce the number of people who become sick with diarrhea by 23 to 40 percent.

The act of not washing your hands can end up harming children. Around 1.8 million children under five will die every year due to pneumonia and diarrheal disease, and these are the top two killers of young children across the world.

Making sure you wash your hands with soap can help to protect about one out of three young children who develop diarrhea, and nearly one out of five young children will become ill with a respiratory infection.

While most people will wash their hands, very few of them actually use soap. Washing hands with soap helps to better remove germs.

Access to soap and handwashing education in school is able to improve attendance.

Having good hand washing techniques early in life can help to improve childhood development in certain settings.

The estimated global rates of washing hands after using the bathroom is only 19 percent.

Washing your hands can also help to battle the rise of antibiotic resistance. When you prevent sickness, it helps to reduce the amount of antibiotics that get prescribed and the likelihood that antibiotic resistance will continue to grow. Hand washing helps to prevent around 30 percent of diarrhea-related illnesses, and around 20 percent of respiratory infections. Antibiotics tend to be prescribed, unnecessarily, for these problems. By making sure you reduce the overall number of infections by making sure you wash your hands can help to lower the odds of overusing antibiotics, which the main cause for antibiotic resistance. Hand washing will also cut down on the odds of getting sick from germs that are resistant to most antibiotics.

Problems With Triclosan

Triclosan was first introduced in 1972 for use as a surgical scrub. Since it has been added to many different products. Triclosan is an antimicrobial chemical that destroys or inhibits the growth of microorganisms like fungi or bacteria. When hospitals first began using it in the 70's, it was a great thing because it helped to keep medical instruments sterile. However, with its rapid increase in use, it has become ubiquitous.

Triclosan has been used in many different products, including dish detergent, personal care products, deodorant, cosmetics, toothpaste, soaps, toys, and even clothes. That is a pretty long list of items when it was originally meant for hospital use. It was marketed under the name "Microban," and it promised to keep household items free of bacteria. They even made socks with it, promising that they would keep your feet odor free.

The problem is, triclosan is a known endocrine disruptor and a possible carcinogen. There is a lot of evidence to suggest that the overuse of triclosan has contributed to bacterial resistance. Plus, the fact that it is getting washed down our drains could mean that it is affecting our water as well.

It is also considered a lipophilic, meaning it can accumulate within the body for extended periods of time, and it is detectable in human breast milk, urine, and blood. They found in animal studies that triclosan can alter your hormone regulation. In human health, triclosan is connected to:

- Reproductive and developmental toxicity
- Uncontrolled cell growth
- Increased chance of developing eczema, allergies, and asthma
- Weakening of the immune system
- Abnormal thyroid hormone and endocrine system signaling

Studies have been performed on mice, and those studies found that triclosan depleted them of bifidobacterium, which is a healthy bacteria that has anti-inflammatory effects. Due to this change in gut health, it could increase a person's risk of colonic inflammation and colon cancer. Some of the first studies performed on triclosan were done at extremely high levels, but the mice studies were done at levels that equaled normal human use.

Luckily, the FDA declared that triclosan, along with 24 other antimicrobial compounds, were not safe for antiseptic products. This meant that companies had to stop using triclosan in their soaps and other healthcare products. That said, it still remains ubiquitous in the US market and is still used in some products like yoga mats, athletic gear, kitchenware, and some building materials. It is famously used in Colgate toothpaste because it prevents gingivitis.

How Long Should You Wash If You're Cooking?

I mentioned earlier that a good length of time for washing your hands is 20 seconds, but let's take a more in depth look at washing times. According to a 2018 report by the USDA, around 97 percent of people do not wash our hands correctly. There was a study done in one workplace, where people were trained to properly wash their hands and use sanitization products, and they found that they had 20 percent fewer sick days.

One question people often have is, do I need to wash longer if I am cooking? When preparing food, you need to be mindful of bacteria. You should wash your hands often, about once every few minutes. However, you do not need to wash your hand for a longer amount of time.

If you follow all of the steps we covered above, washing for 20 seconds should be long enough to thoroughly cleanse your hands from pathogens in the food.

Picking the Best Soap

We already discussed the fact that antibacterial soap isn't any better than non-antibacterial soap because it doesn't kill germs any more efficiently. In fact, the Mayo Clinic has said that antibacterial soap can end up breeding stronger and resilient bacteria.

You can use any bar, liquid, or powder soap that you have available. If you wash your hands as often as you are supposed to, then you should probably look for a soap that is moisturizing or gentle to keep your hands from drying out. Liquid soap tends to be more convenient. And, contrary to popular belief, it is very unlikely for bar soap to transmit bacteria.

Now, if you find that you have run out of soap at home, or a public bathroom is out, you need to still wash your hands. You should still follow the same procedure sans soap.

A study performed in 2011 compared handwashing with and without soap, and they concluded that even though soap is preferable, washing without is still better than not washing your hands at all.

There is also the hand sanitizer option. Hand sanitizers with 60% alcohol or more are great at getting rid of harmful bacteria. However, they don't do well with dissolving oils and dirt from your hands, and they tend not to cleanse your hands as well as properly washing them. When you're in a pinch and don't have quick access to soap and water, having sanitizer on hand is great for getting rid of possible contaminants. That said, if you are taking care of sick loved ones, changing diapers, or cooking, you should wash your hands.

Once you get into the groove of properly washing your hands, it will quickly become second nature. Scrubbing your hands for 20 minutes is enough time for the soap to work its magic and to remove bacteria and other microbes. You should try to be more mindful of washing your hands during flu season, and whenever you are caring for people who have a compromised immune system.

CHAPTER 2: THE BASIC OF HAND SANITIZER

It seems like everywhere you look lately, everyone has a bottle of hand sanitizer readily available. What we want to know is do these little bottles of alcohol based gel actually works to sanitize your hands. We decided to ask a professor about it.

Do Hand Sanitizers Actually Work?

I have always been skeptical about hand sanitizers and never actually thought they worked. Once I did enough research and covered all the bases, I can truthfully say that yes, they actually work. They work very well for most viruses and bacteria. It can kill off the bacteria a lot better than just using soap and water. It can also keep bacteria off the skin longer than just using soap and water. It doesn't damage the skin like soap can because it is made with emollients in it. People who have occupations where they are required to wash their hands a lot usually have problems with their skin drying out and cracking. This can be breeding grounds for bacteria. Hand sanitizers will never replace soap and water completely, but using it along with washing your hands regularly; can help fight all those icky germs.

How it Works?

Hand sanitizers give people an effective and convenient way to clean their hands if they don't have soap and water available as long as their hands aren't covered in visible grease or dirt. Any product can be considered hand sanitizer if its active ingredient is benzalkonium chloride, isopropyl alcohol, or ethyl alcohol.

The FDA hasn't decided to categorize these ingredients as safe since there hasn't been enough research done yet. They aren't pulling these products from the shelves any time soon, either. Other ingredients haven't shown any evidence at being effective in killing germs and haven't been given the FDA's stamp of approval.

Hand sanitizer works by killing cells. It doesn't kill human cells. It only kills microbial cells. Its basis is 70 percent isopropyl alcohol, which is regular rubbing alcohol. This is the best for killing germs. This formula is more effective than the kind that is 100 percent alcohol. Since it has some water in it, it can be absorbed into the skin better. To kill viruses, the sanitizer works by breaking up the virus's outer layer. To kill bacterium, it works by breaking up the cell's membranes. It isn't a cure-all but since some viruses don't have an outer coat or a bacterium that forms spores aren't susceptible.

- Science behind the alcohol

Since the main ingredient in hand sanitizer is alcohol, let's learn more about alcohol. Alcohols are molecules that are made out of hydrogen, oxygen, and carbon. Ethanol is a chemical that is found in alcoholic drinks. It is what most people think of when they say the word alcohol. Isopropanol and propanol better known as isopropyl alcohol, are two more alcohols that can be found commonly in disinfectants since they are easily dissolved in water like ethanol does.

Alcohols kill pathogens that cause diseases by breaking their proteins apart, splitting their cells, or they mess up the cell's metabolism. Products that only have about 30 percent alcohol can still kill some germs but its effectiveness increases with the amount of alcohol that is in the product. Studies show that alcohol can kill various viruses and bacteria if the concentration is more than 60 percent. It will work better as the concentration gets larger. Alcohol's effectiveness stops about 90 percent.

Another good thing about alcohol is bacteria can't develop a resistance to it. Alcohol won't lose its effectiveness the more you use it.

Ethanol is extremely powerful, and some studies have found if used in high concentrations, it can kill three species of bacteria that cause diseases: staphylococcus saprophyticus, serratia marcescens, and Escherichia coli when compared to washing your hands regularly with antibacterial soap.

Alcohol won't work on every germ like the Clostridium difficile or norovirus that could cause diarrhea that can become life threatening or cryptosporidium, which is a parasite that can cause a disease that causes diarrhea called cryptosporidiosis. Hand sanitizers won't remove chemicals like heavy metals or pesticides and they won't work on greasy or dirty hands. In these instances, soap and water are still the best.

Some studies have shown that hand sanitizers that contain benzalkonium chloride as its active ingredient is as effective as and possibly more effective than alcohol when killing bacteria. The benzalkonium chloride needs to be at a concentration of .13 percent to be effective. This hand sanitizer was called HandClens. The scientist that created the product and did all the research worked in a laboratory that has since been closed down. This doesn't mean that it isn't effective; there just hasn't been a lot of research done to find out if it is better than alcohol. Benzalkonium chloride could be harmful to some people in very high concentrations.

The CDC says that hand sanitizers that don't have alcohol might not kill as many germs and could only reduce germs growing rather than killing them completely. To have the best effectiveness against germs, the hand sanitizer needs to have a minimum of 60 percent alcohol.

Is Hand Sanitizer Safe?

Some people think that using hand sanitizer isn't good since it keeps humans from building up a natural resistance to germs. There isn't any evidence for that statement.

Alcohol is safe to be used as an antiseptic and shouldn't have any toxic effects on the skin, but repeated use could cause mild irritation or dryness. Some studies have shown that repeated use is less irritating than constantly washing your hands with soap. If your skin is damaged, the alcohol will probably irritate it more. Which would you rather have some mild irritation or contract or distribute an illness?

Some physicians would tell parents that if they didn't want their children to have an allergy to cats, don't get a cat. Doctors have said this to their patients for the past 50 years. There is more evidence that if you do have cats, you might have protection against some allergies.

This is similar to the statement above, but there just isn't enough evidence to support this idea one way or another.

Does it Work on Preventing the Flu?

This is the best protection for any type of flu strain. Hand sanitizers are very effective in controlling the spread of flu viruses.

Does hand sanitizer only fight against the flu and colds?

Hand sanitizers work on many different viral and bacterial illnesses. Depending on what the bacteria or virus is, it might be less or more susceptible or tolerant to hand sanitizers. For most of what people need to worry about in their daily lives like gastrointestinal and respiratory infections, most viruses or bacteria that cause these illnesses are very susceptible to hand sanitizers.

Should Health Care Workers Use Hand Sanitizers?

If a person works in an environment where they come in contact with humans on a regular basis, they could transfer germs from patient to patient. Anything that works in controlling infections and preventing them will be helpful.

We have always had a problem with health care workers complying with the guidelines of washing their hands often because it is usually very inconvenient to have to stop every few minutes and take the time to wash your hands. Having a bottle of hand sanitizer in every exam room or patient room where a nurse or doctor can pump some in their hand before touching the patient makes it faster and easier than having to go to the sink and wash their hands with soap and water. It can help reduce transmitting germs. Hand sanitizer is a success across the board.

Does it Ever Expire?

Actually, no, hand sanitizer won't ever expire. You will probably see an expiration date on the bottle of sanitizer because the FDA tells the manufacturers that they need to have specific things on the packaging like an expiration date. This date is the last date that the ingredients in the product are supposed to still be effective. It doesn't matter if the manufacturer tested to see how long the product remains safe or if they just came up with a date all on their own. The FDA tells manufacturers to do testing, but not all of them do it.

Alcohol is a chemical that has a long shelf life according to the safety sheet from Sigma Aldrich, which is a chemical supplier. This basically means that if the hand sanitizer is sealed and kept at a steady room temperature, it will remain at the same consistency for a long, long time.

Alcohol can evaporate easily because it has a low boiling point, and after some time, as the bottle gets opened and closed a lot, some of the alcohol could escape out of the bottle, and the concentration might begin to decrease. If you just keep the bottle closed and at a steady room temperature, you will have an effective product for a long, long time.

How and When to Use Sanitizer?

The CDC says you need to wash your hand with soap and water whenever you can since washing your hands can reduce the amount of chemicals and germs on your hands. If you don't have soap and water available, you can use a hand sanitizer to help you stay away from spreading germs and to help you stay healthy. The guide for using hand sanitizer was created based upon the information from many different studies.

Hand sanitizers that are made with a base of alcohol can reduce how many microbes are on your hands, but they won't get rid of every germ. Why can't they kill all germs? Soap and water still tend to kill certain types of germs more efficiently than hands sanitizers. Even though hand sanitizers can make most microbes inactive, they can be effective when used the right way. People might not use enough sanitizer or they might wipe it off before it has time to dry.

Hand sanitizers aren't as effective if your hands are covered in grease or dirt. Why? Well studies have shown that hand sanitizers work great in settings like doctor's offices, hospitals, urgent care centers, etc. where hands touch germs more often, but they won't work on hands that are heavily soiled. Data has shown that it could work on some germs if the hands are only slightly soiled. If hands are very dirty or greasy like after you have handled food, played a sport, worked in your garden, or while fishing or camping, hand sanitizers won't work as well. You absolutely must wash your hands with soap and water.

Hand sanitizers may not remove heavy metals, pesticides, and harmful chemicals from your hands. Even though not many studies have been done about what chemicals hand sanitizers can remove, one study shows that some people who regularly used hand sanitizers had an increased level of pesticides in their bloodstream. If you have touched chemicals that are harmful to you, wash them carefully with soap and water.

If you don't have soap and water readily available, you can use hand sanitizer. Most studies have shown that hand sanitizers that have between 60 and 90 percent alcohol concentration are the best at killing germs than lower concentrations of alcohol. These hand sanitizers might reduce the growth of germs instead of killing them.

When you use hand sanitizer, apply it to the palm of your hand, and then rub the product over all the surfaces of your hand until your hands are completely dry. These steps for use were based on a procedure that was recommended by the CDC. Telling people to completely cover every surface of your hand has been found to give you the best disinfection.

Never swallow hand sanitizer as this can cause alcohol poisoning. Ethyl alcohol based hand sanitizers are safe if you use them as directed, but it could cause alcohol poisoning if you were to swallow a few mouthfuls.

Between the years of 2011 and 2015, the Unites States poison control center received over 85,000 calls about hand sanitizer and children. Children might accidentally swallow hand sanitizers if they are scented, have a bright color, or have an attractive package. Hand sanitizer, just like any other chemical in your home, needs to be stored out of reach of young children. They should only be applied under adult supervision. Using child-resistant caps can reduce poisonings in young children.

Adults and older children may swallow hand sanitizer to try and get drunk.

Five Hidden Dangers

Hand sanitizer has become the new norm for most people these days. You squirt some in your hand. You feel a cooling sensation, and then you rub it onto your hands. Instantly, you feel cleaner.

It sounds like a simpler alternative to using water to wash your hands. It is convenient, portable, and quick, especially if there isn't any clean running water nearby. Hand sanitizer can be found in liquid, foam, or gel forms.

Hand sanitizers normally contain some type of alcohol along with glycerin, fragrance, and water. There are other hand sanitizers that contain compounds that are called triclocarban or triclosan. You can find this ingredient in toothpaste and soaps. These are normally labels as antiseptic, antimicrobial, or antibacterial.

The FDA states that triclosan might carry some unnecessary risks since their risks haven't been proven as of yet.

While using hand sanitizer is perfectly safe, you can end up overusing it. Overuse can expose you to things that can end up harming your body in various ways.

Here are the five dangers that you might not know about:

1. Toxic Chemicals

If you have a scented hand sanitizer, it is probably loaded with chemicals that are toxic. Companies don't have to share the ingredients they use to make their scents, and this means that they could be loaded with a bunch of horrible chemicals.

Phthalates are a common chemical used in many synthetic fragrances. These chemicals disrupt the endocrine system that can change the development of genitals. You should also be on the lookout for parabens. Most skincare products contain these. They are preservatives and can extend the product's life.

2. Antibiotic Resistance

Antibiotics work great in the fight against bacteria. What could happen if your body creates a resistance to said antibiotic and then promotes a resistance to this bacteria?

Triclosan can cause the human body to become resistant to antibiotics. When you use hand sanitizers, you might lower your resistance to certain diseases because you are killing off the good bacteria that is working to protect your body from bad bacteria.

In one study done at the CDC, they found that health care workers who used hand sanitizers more than soap and water were more at risk for getting norovirus, which could lead to acute cases of gastroenteritis.

Being overly exposed to antibiotics or using antibiotics improperly could lead to you becoming bacterial resistant. This will make it harder or close to impossible to treat.

3. Weakened Immune System

Since many hand sanitizers contain triclosan, you need to be careful when using them. As we have already talked about before, triclosan has the ability to harm the immune system. It is important that we maintain a healthy immune system because it is what protects us from diseases.

Researchers have found that triclosan could affect the immune system in a negative way. It can compromise the immune systems to make people more likely to develop allergies, and it can also make them more vulnerable to Bisphenol A, a chemical, which is highly toxic. This can be found in plastics. One this study, teens and children who have high levels of triclosan are diagnosed with allergies and hay fever more often than others.

4. Disruption of Hormones

Another problem with triclosan is problems with your hormones. The FDA states that triclosan might lead to disruptions in hormone production that will cause bacteria to change up the antimicrobial properties it contains. This makes more strains that are resistant to antibiotics. Some research has found that triclosan could end up changing the way our hormones perform their duties. This raises worries and makes more research needed to understand the ways it affects the human body.

5. Alcohol Poisoning

Even if the hand sanitizer doesn't contain triclosan, it does not make it completely safe. Alcohol in the main ingredient in hand sanitizers as it is what kills the bacteria. The FDA and the CDC recommend isopropyl or ethyl alcohol or a mixture of them both with a concentration of at least 60 percent.

During the month of March 2012, six teenagers in California were put in the hospital for alcohol poisoning after they ingested the sanitizer. This made it the latest household product to be used to try and make one drunk. Drinking a couple squirts can equal drinking a few shots of any liquor.

It isn't just teenagers that are doing this; young children have accidentally ingested it, too.

Homemade Hand Sanitizer - Albert Leinstein

Hand sanitizer has its place, and is great to have on hand when you don't have running water nearby, but use it sparingly and keep it out of reach of young children.

CHAPTER 3: HAND SANITIZER RECIPES

We've discussed the necessity of good hygiene and sanitization. That means we need to make sure we have good hand sanitizer on hand whenever we might need, especially in situations where soap and running water isn't available. We're going to take a look at several different hand sanitizer recipes that you can make and keep with you. While you can typically find hand sanitizer in stores, making things from can be more affordable and fun.

As you read through these sanitizer recipes, you will find that there are some that don't use alcohol and makes use of all natural ingredients. All of these recipes will help to cleanse your hands when you need them to, but none of them have been tested in a lab to prove their efficacy against certain diseases, especially the all natural ingredients. If you need to use sanitizer for the purpose of preventing disease, according to the CDC, you should use a hand sanitizer that is at least 60% alcohol. That said, the ones that don't contain alcohol are just as good for a quick hand cleanse when you're not worried about a disease.

Something that you should keep in mind as you make your own sanitizer is the means by which you are making it. You need to make sure that all of the tools you are using have been properly sanitized as well. Otherwise, the entire recipe will be contaminated. To properly sanitize your equipment, you should wash them in warm soapy water thoroughly, then rinse them in clean, running water. You can take this a step further by submerging them in a sanitizing solution. A sanitizing solution would be a gallon of warm water mixed with a tablespoon of unscented chlorine bleach. You would submerge your items in the sanitizing solution, don't let them sit in it for long, and then place them in a clean dish rack to air-dry. Drying them off with a dishtowel would re-contaminate them.

The World Health Organization also suggests once you have made your hand sanitizer, to let it rest for at least 72 hours because this will give the sanitizer a chance to kill any bacteria that may have entered the mixture during the mixing process.

You will also notice that many of these recipes call for essential oils. Purchasing essential oils can be a challenge as there are lots of options on the market, but not all of them are of good quality. It is important that you purchase essential oils that are of high quality, especially for the sanitizers that rely on the anti-microbial powers of the oils. Before we jump into the recipes, I wanted to quickly cover some things about essential oils to make sure you get the best oils for your sanitizers.

Essential oils are a concentrated oil derived from a plant. Most oils are extracted from the plant through cold pressing or steam distillation. The oils are extremely potent, and that's why it is not a good idea to put it directly on your skin without dilution. Essential oils are found in a lot of different things, from incense and perfumes to cosmetics and flavorings.

When it comes to picking out essential oils, the first thing you will want to do is sniff the oil. Now, do not pick up a bottle and just sniff. This can end up causing a headache because the oil is strong. Instead, pick up only the lid, and hold it about five inches from you and sniff. Never place undiluted oil on your skin because you could be allergic. You should also take a break between sniffs as you don't want to overwhelm your senses. This can end up creating difficulty in discerning various fragrant notes.

A good rule of them is to avoid companies that price all of the essential oils at the same price. The extraction process can vary greatly depending on the place, and it would not make sense for agarwood essential oil, which costs about $800 per ounces, to be priced anywhere close to the same price as lemon essential oil, which is about $15 per ounce. Cheap prices suggest that the oil is low quality or synthetic. The price of the oil is based upon the amount of raw material they use.

Also, you should never buy essential oil that has been diluted with vegetable oil. To figure out if it has been diluted, drop a bit on a piece of paper. If it ends up forming an oily ring, then it probably contains vegetable oil. Pick out oils from companies that list their common name and Latin name on the label, along with the country of origin. This will let you know that you are buying the right oil instead of a generically named one. For example, sandalwood oil can come from several different forms of sandalwood.

Real essential oils will always be sold in blue or dark amber glass bottles. Clear glass allows light to enter and cause the oil to go buy. Essential oils should never be sold in plastic containers because undiluted oils can dissolve the plastic and contaminate it. You should also be less rather than more because a 10 ml bottle will normally last several months. If you buy too much, it will probably spoil before you use it.

Typically, oils need to be used within a year, but their shelf life can vary. You can extend their shelf life by keeping them in the refrigerator, but not the freezer.

Hand Sanitizer #1

- Essential oil – this is optional, but you can use a few drops of lavender or tea tree oil

- Vitamin E oil or vegetable glycerin, .5 tsp – optional, but this adds moisturizing properties

- Aloe Vera, 1 tbsp – this keeps the alcohol from drying out your hands

- 190 proof alcohol, 3 tbsp – at least 120 proof, or you can use 70%+ isopropyl rubbing alcohol

To make your hand sanitizer, all you need to do is add everything to a bowl and mix them together. Once they are combined, place the sanitizer into a squeeze tube bottle so that it is easy to use. This recipe will provide you with two fluid ounces of sanitizer.

Natural Hand Sanitizer #1

This homemade hand sanitizer is great because it makes use of all-natural ingredients, and receives all of its wonderful antibacterial and antiviral properties from a cocktail of essential oils. While this particular hand sanitizer has never been tested in a lab for efficacy, it does contain generally accepted anti-microbial ingredients that you should good about using on your hands, and on the hands of those you love.

- Distilled water – or at least filtered, boiled, and cooled
- Tea tree oil, 5 drops
- Orange essential oil, 5 drops
- Lemon essential oil, 5 drops
- Witch hazel with aloe, vodka, or 190 proof alcohol, 3 tbsp
- Vitamin E oil, 5 drops – optional
- 2 oz dark spray bottle

Open up the spray bottle and add the vitamin E oil along with the alcohol or witch hazel, and the essential oils. Screw the lid on and shake the bottle well for 15 to 20 seconds in order to mix everything together.

Open up the bottle again, and fill it the rest of the way with the distilled water. Screw the lid back on and shake for another 15 to 20 seconds. You can print out a label to place on the bottle so that you know exactly what is inside. When you want to use this sanitizer, make sure you shake it first and then spray liberally on your hands and rub together until dry.

Let's take a moment to talk about the ingredients in these particular recipes. Lemon and orange essential oils are both natural disinfectants. It has been proven that tea tree oil can kill fungi, mold, bacteria, and viruses. It also has natural anti-inflammatory properties.

If you tend to be light sensitive, it is best to use this with caution. Both orange and lemon oils can cause photosensitivity, meaning that your skin will be more sensitive to sunlight. The oils in these recipes are very diluted, but it is best to use caution if you are already prone to sunburns. There are many different essential oils out there that have antiseptic properties, so you can always experiment with ones that don't cause photosensitivity.

The witch hazel or alcohol is used to dilute the essential oils, as well as add extra antiseptic properties. Witch hazel is the least anti-microbial of the options in these recipes, but it can also nourish your hands, especially if you choose one with aloe vera in it. Vodka, or any alcohol, is the gold standard for anti-microbial properties. Most vodka that you can find in stores is about 40 to 45 percent alcohol, which is 80 to 90 proof. This recipe will then further dilute. This makes it a "middle of the road" sanitizer. If you want to go to the highest anti-microbial properties, then you would need to use high proof grain alcohol, such as Everclear 190. It is 95% alcohol undiluted, and once mixed into this recipe puts the percentage at 70 to 75. This tends to be very drying.

Hand Sanitizer #2

- Essential oils, 10 drops – lavender oil is a good option, or you can use plain lemon juice
- Aloe Vera gel, .25 c
- Isopropyl alcohol, .75 c

Add everything into a bowl and mix everything together. You can then use a whisk to beat it all together so that it turns into a gel. An electric hand mixer may be easier to use. Using a funnel, pour the mixture into empty squeeze bottles for easy use. Label the bottles with hand sanitizer so that they don't accidentally get used for something else.

Hand Sanitizer #3

- Tea tree oil
- Aloe Vera gel, 3 tbsp
- Isopropyl alcohol, 9 tbsp

All you need to do is mix together the aloe and the alcohol together and then add in a few drops of the tea tree oil to give it a bit of a better scent. It also adds in some anti-microbial properties. Pour into a squeeze or pump bottle and label. You can adjust the size of this recipe easily. All you need to do is make sure that you have a 3:1 ratio of alcohol to aloe vera gel.

Hand Sanitizer #4

- Spray bottle
- Distilled water, 3 oz
- Hydrogen peroxide, 1 tbsp
- Glycerin or glycerol, 1 tsp
- Isopropyl alcohol, 12 oz

Most of the recipes we have gone through are gels, and while they work well, they do tend to leave your hands sticky, which can get annoying. This is a spray hand sanitizer, and has a stronger potency than any other hand sanitizer recipe we have gone over or will go over. It is created based on the recommendations by the World Health Organization. Also, the glycerol is used in this recipe to make sure that you don't dry your hands out with the alcohol. You can typically find it fairly easily online, but if you can't get any to use in this recipe, simply make sure that you moisturize your hands after using this sanitizer.

Alright, begin by mixing together the alcohol with the glycerol until well combined. Stir in the hydrogen peroxide along with the distilled water. If you don't have distilled water, you can also boil tap water and allow it to cool before using it. If you don't have the highest concentration of isopropyl alcohol, don't use as much water because you want to keep the alcohol's potency.

Then pour the mixture into some spray bottles. When you need to use it, spray it onto your hands and rub them together until dry. You can also use this as a cleaning spray in a pinch.

Hand Sanitizer #5

- 190 proof alcohol, 3 to 4 tbsp
- Lemon essential oil, 6 drops
- Spruce essential oil, 10 drops
- Tea tree essential oil, 20 drops
- Vegetable glycerin, .5 tsp

Place the essential oils and the glycerin into a two ounce glass spray bottle. Shake everything together and then add enough alcohol into the bottle until it is nearly full. Screw the lid back on and shake until everything is well combined. Before you use the sanitizer, shake the bottle gently and spray on hands. Rub them together until they are dry.

Natural Hand Sanitizer #2

- Germ destroyer essential oil, 20 drops

- Aloe Vera gel, .25 c

Wisk the two ingredients together until well combined and then pour into a reusable silicone tube. Use whenever you need to.

You may not have heard of germ destroyer essential oil, but it is a fairly popular essential oil blend among people who like to use green cleaners. The essential oil blend includes organic lemon for a burst of energy, organic marjoram and organic lavender for relaxation, and organic spruce hemlock and organic Rosalina for congestion. The essential oil blend can be used for other purposes as well. Some people like mix into with a carrier oil and rubbing it on their child's chest as a natural decongestant. It can also be mixed into a cleaning spray to disinfect your home. If you don't want to purchase the actual blend, you can simply add a few drops of each of the essential oils mentioned earlier.

Natural Hand Sanitizer #3

- Vitamin E oil, 1 tsp

- Witch hazel, isopropyl, or grain alcohol, 2 oz

- Aloe vera gel, 1 oz

- Tea tree oil, 25 drops

- Lemongrass essential oil, 6 drops

- Lavender essential oil, 10 drops
- Glass spray bottle, 2 oz

This recipe makes enough sanitizer to fill two two-ounce bottles.

Add the vitamin E oil and the essential oils into a small glass container or bowl and swirl them together to mix. Add in the alcohol or witch hazel and swirl everything together once more. Pour this into the aloe vera gel and mix everything together very well.

Transfer the mixture into clean spray bottles. Using colored bottles will help to protect your essentials from sunlight. This is a great sanitizer to take with you when traveling and can easily be thrown into a backpack or purse. Make sure that you shake gently before you use it.

You can also mix this up and pout into a pump bottle to keep in your home. When you use alcohol and vitamin E, the sanitizer should last for several months because they act as preservatives.

Natural Hand Sanitizer #4

- Vitamin E oil, 1 tsp
- Aloe Vera gel, 3 tbsp
- Rubbing alcohol or witch hazel, 1 tbsp

- Essential oil, 3 drops – you want essential oils with purifying properties. These include thieves blend, eucalyptus, rosemary, cinnamon, clove, peppermint, thyme, or lavender
- Tea tree essential oil, 2 drops

All you need to do to make this hand sanitizer is to pour all of the ingredients into a bowl and mix them together. Then pour the mixture into a squeeze tube, and you're done. You may want to shake the sanitizer a bit before using it as the essential oils have a tendency to separate.

3 in 1 Hand Sanitizer

- Distilled water
- Tea tree oil
- Aloe Vera gel

For this recipe, you get to choose which type of sanitizer you want; gel, lotion, or liquid. If you want a gel sanitizer, you will need a squeeze tube. Liquid sanitizers will need a spray bottle, and the lotion works well in pump bottles. If you want to be able to carry them with you, you will want bottles that are four to six ounces in size. Each type will use a variation of the ingredients listed above.

For the gel hand sanitizer, you will use only the aloe vera gel and the tea tree oil. If you don't want it to be sticky, make sure you by a high-quality aloe vera gel, and make sure it is 100% aloe. Take your squeeze tube and fill it almost all of the way full with the aloe gel. Add in two to eight drops of the tea tree oil. How much oil you use will depend on what quality your oil is. Mix them together and screw on the lid.

For the liquid hand sanitizer, you will use only the tea tree oil and the distilled water. Begin by filling your spray bottle with distilled water. For a bottle, four to six ounces, you will need to add about two to eight drops of the tea tree oil, depending on the quality of your oil. Shake to combine. You will need to shake this before using it.

For the lotion sanitizer, you will use all three ingredients. Fill up your bottle halfway with the distilled water. Add in some aloe, mixing after each addition, until it reaches the consistency as you like. You can add more water if you need to. Once again, mix in two to eight drops of the tea tree oil. If you are using a larger pump bottle for your lotion, you will need to use more tea tree oil.

Hand Sanitizer #6

- Lavender essential oil, 2 drops
- Clove essential oil, 2 drops
- Cinnamon essential oil, 4 drops

- Orange essential oil, 4 drop
- Alcohol, .66 c
- Witch hazel, 1 oz
- Aloe Vera gel, .33 c

As always, you need to make sure that the alcohol you are using is 60% or more, and this is why most people like to use Everclear grain alcohol or 99% rubbing alcohol. Mix all of your ingredients together and then pour into a squeeze bottle.

CHAPTER 4: HOMEMADE DISINFECTANT WIPES

Companies like to make us think that we need wipes for every single thing we have in our houses like babies' bottoms, faces, toilets, countertops, faucets, etc. I will be the first to admit I used to buy these wipes all the time. I had a container of these under every sink. They sat in their spot right beside other chemical cleaners and the paper towels.

I woke up one day and realized that these were very wasteful, and I spent a lot of money on them over the years. What happened to using a sponge, old washcloth, or old rag to clean and disinfect the counters? Those days have long since died out after companies figured out how to manufacture wipes full of all sorts of chemicals that are harmful to our health. They made them fast and convenient and we didn't have to think about it. These companies can't make any money if we take our wallets back and learn how to make our own disinfecting wipes.

Some of the recipes you will find below use paper towels, which are just being thrown away, too, but the difference is you are making them with healthy cleaners that won't harm your family or pets. Other recipes will use reusable materials like old socks that don't have mates, cut up tee shirts, cut up sheets, old washcloths, etc.

No Need for Commercial Wipes

Most people will spend more than 70 dollars on cleaning wipes each year. These are packaged in plastic and eventually thrown into the trash. You have the choice of whether you want to use paper towels or old rags to make your wipes.

Other than being extremely expensive, wipes that you buy from the store are full of harmful chemicals, such as bleach as their disinfectant. Yes, bleach does kill germs, but it has a lot of harmful side effects that these companies have known about for years.

Why not make your own cleaning wipe that is going to disinfect your house with all-natural ingredients like essential oils, vinegar, and grain alcohol. If you want a wipe that can be reused, find an old sock, tee shirts, sheets, washcloths, etc. that you can repurpose for them?

Homemade wipes are very easy to make, and they will save you tons of money in the long run. Most of the recipes below will leave your surfaces shiny and won't hurt your loved ones. If you don't like the essential oil that a recipe lists, by all means, change it out for one you do like.

Cleaning Versus Disinfecting

Most people don't know that there is a difference between disinfecting and cleaning. When you disinfect, you are killing germs and viruses on objects and surfaces. When you clean, you are getting rid of impurities, liquids, food, and dirt from surfaces.

Most of the homemade wipe recipes out there are great for everyday cleaning, but they aren't the best disinfectant. If you want to make an effective disinfecting wipe, the solution needs to be made from alcohol that is no less than 70 percent pure alcohol such as grain alcohol, that is 140 proof or isopropyl alcohol which is better known as rubbing alcohol.

It is easy to make disinfectant wipes that don't contain harsh chemicals; all you need is a good recipe, and we've got you covered.

Three Most Common Ingredients

- Alcohol

Alcohol is a natural antiviral and antibacterial. You might be wondering how alcohol can kill bacteria and viruses. Alcohol causes damage to the organisms' cell walls. This lets the alcohol enter that organism and essentially destroys them.

The CDC recommends that you use alcohol that is no less than 70 percent pure alcohol. You can either use isopropyl alcohol (rubbing alcohol) or ethanol (grain alcohol). Both of these are great disinfectants. Here are some alcohols that can be used to make a great disinfectant for surfaces to kill germs and viruses.

You need to look for ethanol products that are at least 140 proof or higher. These are all drinkable alcohols. You can find these in your local liquor store.

- Golden Grain: 95 percent alcohol, 190 proof

- Spirytus Vodka: Most of the vodka that is sold in the US is only about 40 percent or 80 proof. If you can find Spirytus Vodka, it is 96 percent alcohol or 192 proof. When you use vodka in your disinfecting wipes, be sure you choose one that is no less than 140 proof.

- Everclear: 92.4 percent alcohol, 190 proof

You need to look for isopropyl alcohol products in the pharmacy section of your local stores.

Find bottles that are labeled as isopropyl alcohol. You can find different percentages:

- 99 percent rubbing alcohol
- 91 percent rubbing alcohol
- 70 percent rubbing alcohol

* Essential Oil

There are several essential oils that have antimicrobial, antiseptic, antifungal, deodorizing, antibacterial, and antiviral properties. When essential oils are used the right way, they can be great at killing germs, and they are safe to be used around small children. When you combine essential oils, they could give you enough protection to kill pathogens like salmonella, MRSA, and E. coli. Essential oils are an amazing product. They are good for so many different things. The ones listed below would be great to use in any disinfecting wipe.

1. Peppermint: antiviral, antibacterial, antiseptic

2. Thyme: antiseptic, antimicrobial, antifungal, antiviral, antibacterial

3. Clove: antifungal, antibacterial, antiseptic, antiviral

4. Cinnamon: antiseptic, antimicrobial, antiviral, antifungal, antibacterial

5. Rosemary: antimicrobial, antifungal, antibacterial, antiseptic

6. Eucalyptus: antimicrobial, antiseptic, antiviral, antifungal, antibacterial

7. Orange: antifungal, antiviral, antiseptic

8. Lemon: antifungal, antiviral, antiseptic, antimicrobial

9. Geranium: antiseptic, antiviral, antifungal, antibacterial

10. Lavender: antimicrobial, antifungal, antibacterial, antiviral, antiseptic

11. Tea tree: antibacterial, antiviral, antiseptic, antimicrobial, antifungal

- Hydrogen peroxide

Studies have shown that viruses can be inactivated with disinfectant wipes that contain .5 percent hydrogen peroxide if it is mixed with alcohol.

- Vinegar and Castile Soap Aren't Friends

Vinegar is great to be used to clean and disinfect surfaces. Many recipes for disinfecting wipes use vinegar as the main disinfectant. If a recipe calls for Castile soap along with vinegar, they won't work well together. Vinegar is acidic while the soap is basic. They are going to react against each other and cancel the other out. The vinegar will actually turn the soap back into its original oily form. You are going to have a white, curdles, oily, gross product that won't do anything. but soap and vinegar won't mix when making disinfectant wipes.

Where to Use Wipes

These disinfecting wipes can be used in any room in your home and on most surfaces. The surface needs to be hard and non-porous.

Outside

- Airplanes: seatback, tray table, seat belt, air vent
- Restaurant tables
- Shopping carts
- Gearshift and steering wheels in cars

Around the Home

- Doorknobs
- Light switches
- Thermometers
- Phones

- Computer mouse, keyboard, screen
- Remote controls

Bathroom

- Countertops
- Faucets
- Toilet
- Light switches
- Doorknobs
- Tubs

Kitchen

- Oven handle
- Stove knobs
- Refrigerator handle
- Light switches
- Faucet
- Cabinet pulls
- Trashcan
- Countertops

Any of the below recipes could be doubled. Most of these are using a roll of paper towels that have been cut in half. If you double the recipe, you can make two containers of wipes at one time.

Disinfecting Wipe #1

- Rosemary oil, 5 drops
- Eucalyptus oil, 5 drops
- Cinnamon oil, 10 drops
- Clove oil, 15 drops
- Lemon oil, 20 drops
- Hydrogen peroxide, .75 tsp
- Alcohol of choice, 3 c

Put all of the above ingredients into a large pitcher or measuring cup and mix well.

Find a container that has an airtight lid. It needs to be either stainless steel or glass so they won't dilute the essential oils. Some plastics like plastic #2 PET or plastic #1 HDPE will also work well. The container needs to be large enough to hold at least 30 to 40 paper towels along with the disinfecting solution.

Once you have your container, pour two cups of the solution into it.

Now you want to get your paper towels ready. You can use any disposable guest towels, dinner napkins, or paper towels. Just be sure that whatever you pick is a high-quality paper that is fairly thick so that it can stand up to being used.

Use around 30 to 40 "select-a-size" towels. If you are using paper towels, fold each one in half. Then stack them on top of one another. Now place them into your container.

Gently turn the container on its side and move it around so the towels can absorb the liquid.

Pour the rest of the solution into the container. Make sure all of your wipes get wet. There should be some solution in the bottom of your container. This keeps the wipes wet.

Make sure to put a label on your container.

To use your wipes: make sure the surface has been cleaned of any visible dirt. Take a wipe out of your containers and make sure it is wet. Wipe the surface you want to disinfect until you can see it is wet. Allow the surface to dry naturally.

Disinfecting Wipe #2

- Scissors
- Needle

Homemade Hand Sanitizer - Albert Leinstein

- Spray paint (optional)
- Essential oil of choice, 10 drops
- Liquid dish soap, 1 tsp
- Rubbing alcohol, .25 c
- Water, .25 c
- Vinegar, .5 c
- Sharp knife
- Roll of paper towels
- Coffee canister with lid

The above ingredients won't cost you much money, and this means you can make these and have them in every room of your house. Vinegar is great at cleaning plus it kills bacteria, mold, and germs. You can use whatever dish soap you normally use.

You can paint the old coffee can if you would like. It is totally up to you.

To make the wipes, cut the paper towels in half using a knife. A serrated knife works better. Push them down into the can.

Now, mix the water, rubbing alcohol, dish soap, and vinegar together in a bowl. You have the choice to add some essential oil to your wipes if you would like.

Pour the liquid slowly over the towels. When they have become totally saturated, you can remove the centerpiece of cardboard. This allows you to pull the paper towels up from the middle.

Push the needle through the center of the lid a couple of times and then take the scissors and cut an X in the middle. Now you can feed the paper towels up through the X and secure the lid on the can. If the wipes begin to dry out, add a bit more water.

Use it as you will.

Reusable Disinfecting Wipes #3

- Glass jar with a sealable lid
- 10 old washcloths
- Lemon oil, 10 drops
- Dawn dish soap
- Rubbing alcohol, .75 c
- Distilled water, 3 c

If you have clean tap water, by all means, use it to save you some money. Otherwise, they could leave marks on your surfaces that you are trying to clean.

You need to decide how large you would like your wipes. If they are normal-sized washcloths, it would be best to cut them in half. If you have larger surfaces, you can leave some of them whole. Add the washcloths to the jar.

Mix the lemon oil, alcohol, dish soap, and water in a bowl. Pour this mixture over the washcloths. Put the lid on the jar and use it as you need them.

When the cloths get dirty, just throw the dirty clots into the washing machine to give them a good cleaning. Make more solution and carry on.

Disinfecting Wipes #4

You can put your wipes in an old baby wipe container or plastic container if you would like to have them within reach. You could also place this solution into a spray bottle and just spray it on your surfaces and wipe them down.

- Old washcloths or rags of choice
- Ammonia, 2 tbsp
- Dawn dish soap, 1 tsp
- Rubbing alcohol, .25 c
- Water, 1 c

Cut the washcloths or material into squares that measure four inches by six inches. If the washcloths are fairly small, they will probably not need to be cut down.

Mix all the ingredients together and pour over the rags. You might have to adjust the amount you make depending on how many rags you have. You want to make sure you have enough solution to get all of the rags wet. If you make more solution that won't fit in your container, just store it in a spray bottle and use it as a spray cleaner.

Once the rags get dirty, just wash them in the washing machine to be reused.

Disinfecting Wipes #5

- Dish soap, 1 tbsp
- Rubbing alcohol, 1 c
- Warm water, 2 c

Take a roll of paper towels and cut them in half. Place these into a plastic container and pour the mixture over the towels. When the towels are wet, you should be able to pull the cardboard center out so the wipes will pull out from the center.

Disinfecting Wipe #6

- Lemon oil, 35 drops

- Tea tree oil, 30 drops
- Distilled water, 1.5 c
- Castile soap, 3 tbsp
- Vodka, .5 c
- Whatever type of rag or cloth you want to use

Mix the oils, water, soap, and alcohol together in a bowl.

Put some of your cloths into a glass container and pour a little bit of the solution on it.

Keep repeating this process until all of your cloths have absorbed all of the solution.

Place the lid on the container and swirl it around to make sure everything is completely saturated with the solution.

When you are ready to use your wipes, take one out of the container, and wring any excess solution back into the container. Wipe it over the surface you want to disinfect in your home.

Do not reuse your cloths. Put these aside to be laundered normally.

Disinfecting Wipe #7

- Roll of paper towels
- Tea tree oil, 3 drops
- Dawn dish soap, 1 tbsp
- Isopropyl alcohol, 1 c
- Water, 2 c

Take your roll of paper towels and cut them in half using a serrated knife.

Place them into your container of choice. An empty container of wipes works great.

Put the water, alcohol, dish soap, and tea tree oil into a bowl and mix well.

Gently pour this around the center of the paper towel roll until the cardboard is wet. Keep pouring until you can easily pull the cardboard out of the middle of the paper towels.

Pull the towels up from the center and place the lid back on.

Keep in an airtight container that is tightly closed.

Disinfecting Wipes #8

- Simple clean oil, 20 drops**
- Dawn dish soap, 1 tsp
- Rubbing alcohol, .25 c

- Distilled water, 2 c
- Old rags or cloths, clean
- Quart mason jar

Put the essential oil, dish soap, rubbing alcohol, and water into the quart jar. Place the lid on the jar and gently shake it to mix.

Take the lid off the jar and add in the cloths or rags. Continue to add until all the solution has been absorbed and then add in one additional cloth.

Put the lid on the jar and turn the jar upside down for a couple of minutes.

Your wipes are ready to be used.

Just like with any disinfectant wipe, use them on any surface of your choice. Place the used wipes in a basket, or another container until you are ready to wash them. Make another batch of the solution, wash your cloths, and continue to use.

If you have a pile of socks without mates, they will work great as a disinfecting wipe.

**Simple Clean essential oil blend is a mixture of tea tree, pine, sweet orange, cypress, balsam fir, lemongrass, cedarwood, and lemon essential oils. If you can't find simple clean or don't want to buy it, you could just mix the oils listed here and make your own.

Disinfecting Wipes #9

- Roll of paper towels
- Orange oil, 10 drop
- Dawn dish soap, 1 tbsp
- Isopropyl alcohol, 1.25 c
- Distilled water, 2 c

Find an empty wipe container or another container that is large enough for a paper towel roll to fit into.

Cut the roll of paper towels in half using a large serrated knife. Place this inside the container.

Mix together the dish soap, alcohol, essential oil in a bowl. Slowly pour this mixture over the cardboard center of the towels. Once it is wet enough, you can pull the cardboard out.

This should allow you to pull the paper towels up from the center.

Disinfecting Spray

- Spray bottle
- Essential oils of choice

- Alcohol, rubbing or 190 proof grain alcohol

Pour the alcohol into your spray bottle.

Add about 10 drops of every essential oil you want to use. Look back at the list above to pick the ones with the best disinfecting qualities.

Now, shake, shake, shake!

That's it. You're done. Spray on any surface you want to disinfect and wipe with a cloth or paper towel.

If you have a large spray bottle, just pour in alcohol to the desired amount you want to make. Add enough essential oil to make the alcohol smell go away.

Reusable Disinfecting Wipes #11

- Lavender oil, 5 drops
- Tea tree oil, 5 drops
- Rubbing alcohol, .5 c
- Liquid Castile soap, 1 tbsp
- Distilled water, 1 c
- Empty baby wipe container

- Old washcloths, cut up cloths, or socks without a mate

Fold all the socks, cloths, or washcloths and put them inside the container.

Take a glass measuring cup and pour in the essential oils, rubbing alcohol, Castille soap, and water. Whisk to mix well.

Pour on the cloths until they are all wet. Keep the lid on and use it when needed.

Don't put used cloths back into the mixture as this will contaminate the solution. Set the used ones to the side until you are ready to wash them and make a new batch of disinfectant.

When ready to wash, simply wash in your washing machine like you would anything else.

Reusable Disinfecting Wipes #12

- 10 X 10 pieces of old tee shirts, 15 to 20
- Mason jar, quart, wide-mouth, with lid
- Bergamot oil, 4 drops
- Lavender oil, 8 drops
- Lemon oil, 15 drops
- White vinegar, .75 c

- Distilled water, .75 c

Place all of the liquid ingredients into the mason jar, place the lid on and swirl to combine.

Fold the pieces of cloth and place them into the liquid. Press each one firmly so it can soak up the solutions. Place the lid on tightly and turn the jar upside down to make sure everything is soaked through.

Store in a dark, cool place to preserve the essential oils.

When ready to use, take one cloth out of the jar and wring out excess liquid. After you have used the cloth, rinse with cool water and set to the side until ready to launder.

Disinfecting Spray

We've gone over lots of recipes for disinfectant wipes, but I've got one last disinfectant for you. This is a disinfectant spray that you can use to disinfect your home after you have cleaned. This is a spray that you can spray on everything in your home, including your sofa, bed, and pillows. It does not need to be wiped up. Simply spray it on, let it dry, and the surface is not, temporarily, cleaned of germs.

- Tea tree essential oil, 5 to 60 drops – you can also use lavender essential oil if you would prefer

- White distilled vinegar, .5 c

- 100 proof alcohol, 1.5 c – you can use a higher proof alcohol if you would like, you can get Everclear 190. You do not, however, want to use rubbing alcohol as it can damage varnished or painted surfaces.

Using a 16-ounce spray bottle, pour the alcohol in and followed by the essential oils. Screw on the lid and shake the bottle to combine the alcohol and oils. Open the bottle back up and add in the vinegar. Shake the bottle once more to combine everything together. Since it contains vinegar, you should avoid using this spray on stone surfaces, such as marble and granite. If you have stone surfaces in your home, you can simply add an extra ½ cup of alcohol to the recipe.

Shake the bottle well before you use the disinfectant.

Keep in mind that 100 proof alcohol is not the same thing as 100% alcohol. 100 proof is only 50% alcohol, and is the minimum you should use in any disinfectant recipe.

CONCLUSION

Thank you for making it through to the end of *Homemade Hand Sanitizer*, let's hope it was informative and able to provide you with all of the tools you need to achieve your goals whatever they may be.

It is important every day to practice good hygiene. In doing so, it helps to reduce your chances of getting sick and reduces the spread of communicable diseases. Be sure you do your part by making sure you are clean and in doing so, won't spread any disease.

This book is here to help you with that by providing you with information on basic hygiene and sanitization. The first thing we have gone over is basic hygiene.

The next step is to go grab you some ingredients for your homemade hand sanitizer. It never hurts to always have some hand sanitizer on hand whenever you feel you need a little cleaning up. It is possible to overuse sanitizer, so make sure you use it wisely and sparingly. You can always refresh your memory on sanitizer safety by rereading this book. It can dry out your hands, and if your hands are physically dirty, remember to wash them with soap and water. Sanitizer only sanitizes, it doesn't clean the way soap and water does.

Above all, use common sense when it comes to hygiene and preventing the spread of communicable diseases. The first step begins with you.

Finally, if you found this book useful in any way, a review on Amazon is always appreciated!

www.ingramcontent.com/pod-product-compliance
Lightning Source LLC
Chambersburg PA
CBHW071146240526
45465CB00024BA/1801